Introduction

Welcome to the "Dementia Caregiver's Daily Journal — Charting the Heart's Journey: A Year of Reflection, Resilience, and Rediscovery"—your compassionate companion on the deeply personal and challenging journey of caring for a loved one with dementia. As a caregiver, you play an essential role not only in the life of the person with dementia but in the broader tapestry of humanity. Your dedication, love, and unwavering commitment deserve recognition and support.

Dementia caregiving is a multifaceted role that brings with it a myriad of emotions—joy, sorrow, frustration, hope, and everything in between. This journal offers a sacred space to express your feelings, document daily experiences, and reflect on the lessons and memories you're creating.

Structure of the Journal:

The journal comprises 52 series, mirroring the weeks in a year.
Each series includes:

Seven Journal Pages: Each day, you will have a space to record moments, both challenging and heartwarming. Here, you can note your observations, vent frustrations, celebrate small victories, or simply ponder your feelings. It's your personal canvas—fill it as you see fit.

Mental Health Check-in Page: At the end of every seven journal pages, there's a specially designed page for you to 'check in' with yourself. As a caregiver, you often prioritize your loved one's well- being over your own. This page serves as a gentle reminder that your mental health is paramount. By regularly assessing and acknowledging your emotions, you can take proactive steps to seek support or make necessary changes in your routine.

I understand that each day with dementia is unpredictable. You may feel a profound connection some days, while others might be more trying. Regardless of the day's nature, know that this journal is here to provide a listening ear.

As you navigate the intricate dance of dementia caregiving, let this journal serve as a testament to your resilience, love, and dedication. Remember, in the intricate web of caregiving, your story matters, too. By chronicling your journey, you not only aid in your personal healing and reflection but also inspire and guide others who embark on a similar path.

Wishing you strength, peace, and moments of unexpected joy in your caregiving journey.

G. M. Grace

DEMENTIA CAREGIVER'S DAILY JOURNAL

CHARTING THE HEART'S JOURNEY: A YEAR OF REFLECTION, RESILIENCE, AND REDISCOVERY

G.M. GRACE

AUTHOR OF

DEMENTIA CAREGIVER'S
PRACTICAL GUIDE

Daily Journal

Date:

Daily Journal

Date:

Daily Journal

Date:

Daily Journal

Date:

Daily Journal

Date:

Daily Journal

Date:

Daily Journal

Date:

Weekly check in

DATE____________

TOP 3 THINGS I DID THIS WEEK

○ _______________________
○ _______________________
○ _______________________

THIS WEEK I FELT

NEXT WEEK I WANT TO

MOST REWARDING INTERACTION I HAD THIS WEEK

THINGS I ACCOMPLISHED THIS WEEK

WHAT WAS THE BEST THING ABOUT THE WEEK?

MY RANKING OF THE WEEK

☆ ☆ ☆ ☆ ☆

Daily Journal

Date:

Daily Journal

Date:

Daily Journal

Date:

Daily Journal

Date:

Daily Journal

Date:

Daily Journal

Date:

Daily Journal

Date:

Weekly check in

DATE _______________

TOP 3 THINGS I DID THIS WEEK _______________

- ☐
- ☐
- ☐

THIS WEEK I FELT

MOST REWARDING INTERACTION I HAD THIS WEEK

NEXT WEEK I WANT TO _______________

THINGS I ACCOMPLISHED THIS WEEK

WHAT WAS THE BEST THING ABOUT THE WEEK?

MY RANKING OF THE WEEK

Your Next Essential Read
"Dementia Caregiver's Practical Guide"

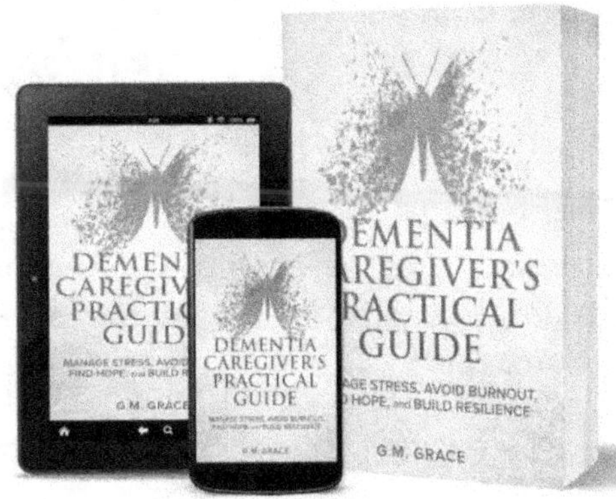

Are you looking to delve deeper into the world of dementia caregiving? To further equip yourself with practical knowledge, insights, and tools that can make your caregiving journey smoother?

We're delighted to introduce the "Dementia Caregiver's Practical Guide: Manage Stress, Avoid Burnout, Find Hope, and Build Resilience" — a comprehensive resource tailored for caregivers like you. Whether you're in the initial stages of understanding dementia or have been on this journey for some time, this guide promises valuable insights, techniques, and real-life solutions to the challenges faced by caregivers.

How to Access: We've incorporated a QR code on the next page for your convenience. Scan it with your smartphone or tablet, and it will lead you directly to the purchasing page for the "Dementia Caregiver's Practical Guide: Manage Stress, Avoid Burnout, Find Hope, and Build Resilience."

This seamless process ensures that the next step in your caregiving resource journey is just a scan away.

I genuinely believe in empowering caregivers with the best knowledge and support available. This guide is a testament to that belief. May it serve as a beacon of hope, clarity, and practical wisdom in your journey with your loved one.

Your Feedback Matters to Me!

I hope you are finding value in this journal. Your feedback is crucial to help me and others in this community of caregivers make informed choices. I would be deeply appreciative if you could spare a few minutes to share your thoughts and experiences on Amazon.

How to Leave a Review: Scan the QR code below using your smartphone or tablet's camera. This will direct you straight to the review page on Amazon. Share your honest feedback and rate the journal as per your experience.

[Place QR Code Here]

Your insights not only help future readers/customers but also guide us in our mission to

Daily Journal

Date:

Daily Journal

Date:

Daily Journal

Date:

Daily Journal

Date:

Daily Journal

Date:

Daily Journal

Date:

Daily Journal

Date:

Weekly check in

DATE ________________

TOP 3 THINGS I DID THIS WEEK

☆ ________________

☆ ________________

☆ ________________

THIS WEEK I FELT

NEXT WEEK I WANT TO ________________

____

____

____

____

MOST REWARDING INTERACTION I HAD THIS WEEK

THINGS I ACCOMPLISHED THIS WEEK:

WHAT WAS THE BEST THING ABOUT THE WEEK?

MY RANKING OF THE WEEK

☆ ☆ ☆ ☆ ☆

Daily Journal

Date:

Daily Journal

Date:

Daily Journal

Date:

Daily Journal

Date:

Daily Journal

Date:

Daily Journal

Date:

Daily Journal

Date:

Weekly check in

DATE ___________

TOP 3 THINGS I DID THIS WEEK

- _______________________
- _______________________
- _______________________

THIS WEEK I FELT

NEXT WEEK I WANT TO _______________

____
____
____
____

THINGS I ACCOMPLISHED THIS WEEK

MOST REWARDING INTERACTION I HAD THIS WEEK

WHAT WAS THE BEST THING ABOUT THE WEEK?

MY RANKING OF THE WEEK

☆ ☆ ☆ ☆ ☆

Daily Journal

Date:

Daily Journal

Date:

Daily Journal

Date:

Daily Journal

Date:

Daily Journal

Date:

Daily Journal

Date:

Daily Journal

Date:

Weekly check in

DATE ___________

TOP 3 THINGS I DID THIS WEEK

-
-
-

THIS WEEK I FELT

NEXT WEEK I WANT TO

MOST REWARDING INTERACTION I HAD THIS WEEK

THINGS I ACCOMPLISHED THIS WEEK

WHAT WAS THE BEST THING ABOUT THE WEEK?

MY RANKING OF THE WEEK

Daily Journal

Date:

Daily Journal

Date:

Daily Journal

Date:

Daily Journal

Date:

Daily Journal

Date:

Daily Journal

Date:

Daily Journal

Date:

Weekly check in

DATE _______________

TOP 3 THINGS I DID THIS WEEK

- _______________
- _______________
- _______________

THIS WEEK I FELT

NEXT WEEK I WANT TO _______________

____
____
____
____

MOST REWARDING INTERACTION I HAD THIS WEEK

THINGS I ACCOMPLISHED THIS WEEK

WHAT WAS THE BEST THING ABOUT THE WEEK?

MY RANKING OF THE WEEK

☆ ☆ ☆ ☆ ☆

Daily Journal

Date:

Daily Journal

Date:

Daily Journal

Date:

Daily Journal

Date:

Daily Journal

Date:

Daily Journal

Date:

Daily Journal

Date:

Weekly check in

DATE _______________

TOP 3 THINGS I DID THIS WEEK
- ○ _______________
- ○ _______________
- ○ _______________

THIS WEEK I FELT

NEXT WEEK I WANT TO _______________

____

____

____

MOST REWARDING INTERACTION I HAD THIS WEEK

THINGS I ACCOMPLISHED THIS WEEK

WHAT WAS THE BEST THING ABOUT THE WEEK?

MY RANKING OF THE WEEK

Daily Journal

Date:

Daily Journal

Date:

Daily Journal

Date:

Daily Journal

Date:

Daily Journal

Date:

Daily Journal

Date:

Daily Journal

Date:

Weekly check in

TOP 3 THINGS I DID THIS WEEK

○ ______________________________

○ ______________________________

○ ______________________________

THIS WEEK I FELT

NEXT WEEK I WANT TO

____

____

____

____

MOST REWARDING INTERACTION I HAD THIS WEEK

THINGS I ACCOMPLISHED THIS WEEK

WHAT WAS THE BEST THING ABOUT THE WEEK?

MY RANKING OF THE WEEK

☆ ☆ ☆ ☆ ☆

Daily Journal

Date:

Daily Journal

Date:

Daily Journal

Date:

Daily Journal

Date:

Daily Journal

Date:

Daily Journal

Date:

Daily Journal

Date:

Weekly check in

DATE _______________

TOP 3 THINGS I DID THIS WEEK

○ _______________________________

○ _______________________________

○ _______________________________

THIS WEEK I FELT

NEXT WEEK I WANT TO

____

____

____

____

THINGS I ACCOMPLISHED THIS WEEK

MOST REWARDING INTERACTION I HAD THIS WEEK

WHAT WAS THE BEST THING ABOUT THE WEEK?

MY RANKING OF THE WEEK

☆ ☆ ☆ ☆ ☆

Daily Journal

Date:

Daily Journal

Date:

Daily Journal

Date:

Daily Journal

Date:

Daily Journal

Date:

Daily Journal

Date:

Daily Journal

Date:

Weekly check in

DATE _______________

TOP 3 THINGS I DID THIS WEEK

-
-
-

THIS WEEK I FELT

NEXT WEEK I WANT TO

MOST REWARDING INTERACTION I HAD THIS WEEK

THINGS I ACCOMPLISHED THIS WEEK

WHAT WAS THE BEST THING ABOUT THE WEEK?

MY RANKING OF THE WEEK

Daily Journal

Date:

Daily Journal

Date:

Daily Journal

Date:

Daily Journal

Date:

Daily Journal

Date:

89

Daily Journal

Date:

Daily Journal

Date:

Weekly check in

DATE _______________

TOP 3 THINGS I DID THIS WEEK
- ○ _______________
- ○ _______________
- ○ _______________

THIS WEEK I FELT

NEXT WEEK I WANT TO
____
____
____
____

MOST REWARDING INTERACTION I HAD THIS WEEK

THINGS I ACCOMPLISHED THIS WEEK

WHAT WAS THE BEST THING ABOUT THE WEEK?

MY RANKING OF THE WEEK
☆ ☆ ☆ ☆ ☆

Daily Journal

Date:

Daily Journal

Date:

Daily Journal

Date:

Daily Journal

Date:

Daily Journal

Date:

Daily Journal

Date:

Daily Journal

Date:

Weekly check in

DATE ______________

TOP 3 THINGS I DID THIS WEEK

- _______________________
- _______________________
- _______________________

THIS WEEK I FELT

NEXT WEEK I WANT TO

____
____
____
____

MOST REWARDING INTERACTION I HAD THIS WEEK

THINGS I ACCOMPLISHED THIS WEEK

WHAT WAS THE BEST THING ABOUT THE WEEK?

MY RANKING OF THE WEEK

☆ ☆ ☆ ☆ ☆

Daily Journal

Date:

Daily Journal

Date:

Daily Journal

Date:

Daily Journal

Date:

Daily Journal

Date:

Daily Journal

Date:

Daily Journal

Date:

Weekly check in

DATE ______________

TOP 3 THINGS I DID THIS WEEK

- ○ ______________________
- ○ ______________________
- ○ ______________________

THIS WEEK I FELT

NEXT WEEK I WANT TO ______________

____

____

____

____

MOST REWARDING INTERACTION I HAD THIS WEEK

THINGS I ACCOMPLISHED THIS WEEK

WHAT WAS THE BEST THING ABOUT THE WEEK?

MY RANKING OF THE WEEK

☆ ☆ ☆ ☆ ☆

Daily Journal

Date:

Daily Journal

Date:

Daily Journal

Date:

Daily Journal

Date:

Daily Journal

Date:

Daily Journal

Date:

Daily Journal

Date:

Weekly check in

TOP 3 THINGS I DID THIS WEEK

-
-
-

THIS WEEK I FELT

NEXT WEEK I WANT TO

MOST REWARDING INTERACTION I HAD THIS WEEK

THINGS I ACCOMPLISHED THIS WEEK

WHAT WAS THE BEST THING ABOUT THE WEEK?

MY RANKING OF THE WEEK

Daily Journal

Date:

Daily Journal

Date:

Daily Journal

Date:

Daily Journal

Date:

Daily Journal

Date:

Daily Journal

Date:

Daily Journal

Date:

Weekly check in

DATE _______________

TOP 3 THINGS I DID THIS WEEK

○ _______________________________

○ _______________________________

○ _______________________________

THIS WEEK I FELT

NEXT WEEK I WANT TO _______________

____

____

____

____

MOST REWARDING INTERACTION I HAD THIS WEEK

THINGS I ACCOMPLISHED THIS WEEK

WHAT WAS THE BEST THING ABOUT THE WEEK?

MY RANKING OF THE WEEK

☆ ☆ ☆ ☆ ☆

Daily Journal

Date:

Daily Journal

Date:

Daily Journal

Date:

Daily Journal

Date:

Daily Journal

Date:

Daily Journal

Date:

Daily Journal

Date:

Weekly check in

DATE _______________

TOP 3 THINGS I DID THIS WEEK

○ _______________________________

○ _______________________________

○ _______________________________

THIS WEEK I FELT

NEXT WEEK I WANT TO _______________

____

____

____

____

MOST REWARDING INTERACTION I HAD THIS WEEK

THINGS I ACCOMPLISHED THIS WEEK

WHAT WAS THE BEST THING ABOUT THE WEEK?

MY RANKING OF THE WEEK

☆ ☆ ☆ ☆ ☆

Daily Journal

Date:

Daily Journal

Date:

Daily Journal

Date:

Daily Journal

Date:

Daily Journal

Date:

Daily Journal

Date:

Daily Journal

Date:

Weekly check in

DATE ______________

TOP 3 THINGS I DID THIS WEEK
- ○ _______________________
- ○ _______________________
- ○ _______________________

THIS WEEK I FELT

NEXT WEEK I WANT TO

MOST REWARDING INTERACTION I HAD THIS WEEK

THINGS I ACCOMPLISHED THIS WEEK

WHAT WAS THE BEST THING ABOUT THE WEEK?

MY RANKING OF THE WEEK
☆ ☆ ☆ ☆ ☆

Daily Journal

Date:

Daily Journal

Date:

Daily Journal

Date:

Daily Journal

Date:

Daily Journal

Date:

Daily Journal

Date:

Daily Journal

Date:

Weekly check in

DATE _______________

TOP 3 THINGS I DID THIS WEEK

○ _______________________________

○ _______________________________

○ _______________________________

THIS WEEK I FELT

NEXT WEEK I WANT TO

____

____

____

____

MOST REWARDING INTERACTION I HAD THIS WEEK

THINGS I ACCOMPLISHED THIS WEEK

WHAT WAS THE BEST THING ABOUT THE WEEK?

MY RANKING OF THE WEEK

☆ ☆ ☆ ☆ ☆

Daily Journal

Date:

Daily Journal

Date:

Daily Journal

Date:

Daily Journal

Date:

Daily Journal

Date:

Daily Journal

Date:

Daily Journal *Date:*

Weekly check in

DATE _______________

TOP 3 THINGS I DID THIS WEEK

- ________________________
- ________________________
- ________________________

THIS WEEK I FELT

NEXT WEEK I WANT TO _______________

MOST REWARDING INTERACTION I HAD THIS WEEK

THINGS I ACCOMPLISHED THIS WEEK

WHAT WAS THE BEST THING ABOUT THE WEEK?

MY RANKING OF THE WEEK

Daily Journal

Date:

Daily Journal

Date:

Daily Journal

Date:

Daily Journal

Date:

Daily Journal

Date:

Daily Journal

Date:

Daily Journal

Date:

Weekly check in

TOP 3 THINGS I DID THIS WEEK

○ ______________________

○ ______________________

○ ______________________

THIS WEEK I FELT

NEXT WEEK I WANT TO

MOST REWARDING INTERACTION I HAD THIS WEEK

THINGS I ACCOMPLISHED THIS WEEK

WHAT WAS THE BEST THING ABOUT THE WEEK?

MY RANKING OF THE WEEK

Daily Journal

Date:

Daily Journal

Date:

Daily Journal

Date:

Daily Journal

Date:

Daily Journal

Date:

Daily Journal

Date:

Daily Journal

Date:

Weekly check in

TOP 3 THINGS I DID THIS WEEK

- ○ _______________________________
- ○ _______________________________
- ○ _______________________________

THIS WEEK I FELT

NEXT WEEK I WANT TO

____

____

____

____

MOST REWARDING INTERACTION I HAD THIS WEEK

THINGS I ACCOMPLISHED THIS WEEK

WHAT WAS THE BEST THING ABOUT THE WEEK?

MY RANKING OF THE WEEK

☆ ☆ ☆ ☆ ☆

Daily Journal

Date:

Daily Journal

Date:

Daily Journal

Date:

Daily Journal

Date:

Daily Journal

Date:

Daily Journal

Date:

Daily Journal

Date:

Weekly check in

TOP 3 THINGS I DID THIS WEEK

○
○
○

THIS WEEK I FELT

NEXT WEEK I WANT TO

MOST REWARDING INTERACTION I HAD THIS WEEK

THINGS I ACCOMPLISHED THIS WEEK

WHAT WAS THE BEST THING ABOUT THE WEEK?

MY RANKING OF THE WEEK

Daily Journal

Date:

Daily Journal

Date:

Daily Journal

Date:

Daily Journal

Date:

Daily Journal

Date:

Daily Journal

Date:

Daily Journal

Date:

Weekly check in

DATE ___________

TOP 3 THINGS I DID THIS WEEK
- ___________
- ___________
- ___________

THIS WEEK I FELT

NEXT WEEK I WANT TO
____
____
____
____

THINGS I ACCOMPLISHED THIS WEEK

MOST REWARDING INTERACTION I HAD THIS WEEK

WHAT WAS THE BEST THING ABOUT THE WEEK?

MY RANKING OF THE WEEK
☆ ☆ ☆ ☆ ☆

Daily Journal

Date:

Daily Journal

Date:

Daily Journal

Date:

Daily Journal

Date:

Daily Journal

Date:

Daily Journal

Date:

Daily Journal

Date:

Weekly check in

DATE________________

<u>TOP 3 THINGS I DID THIS WEEK</u>

○ _______________________

○ _______________________

○ _______________________

<u>THIS WEEK I FELT</u>

<u>NEXT WEEK I WANT TO</u>

<u>MOST REWARDING INTERACTION I HAD THIS WEEK</u>

<u>THINGS I ACCOMPLISHED THIS WEEK</u>

<u>WHAT WAS THE BEST THING ABOUT THE WEEK?</u>

<u>MY RANKING OF THE WEEK</u>

Daily Journal

Date:

Daily Journal

Date:

Daily Journal

Date:

Daily Journal

Date:

Daily Journal

Date:

Daily Journal

Date:

Daily Journal

Date:

Weekly check in

TOP 3 THINGS I DID THIS WEEK

○ ______________________

○ ______________________

○ ______________________

THIS WEEK I FELT

NEXT WEEK I WANT TO ______________

____

____

____

____

MOST REWARDING INTERACTION I HAD THIS WEEK

THINGS I ACCOMPLISHED THIS WEEK

WHAT WAS THE BEST THING ABOUT THE WEEK?

MY RANKING OF THE WEEK

☆ ☆ ☆ ☆ ☆

Daily Journal

Date:

Daily Journal

Date:

Daily Journal

Date:

Daily Journal

Date:

Daily Journal

Date:

Daily Journal

Date:

Daily Journal

Date:

Weekly check in

DATE _______________

TOP 3 THINGS I DID THIS WEEK _______________

○ _______________

○ _______________

○ _______________

THIS WEEK I FELT

NEXT WEEK I WANT TO _______________

____

____

____

____

MOST REWARDING INTERACTION I HAD THIS WEEK

THINGS I ACCOMPLISHED THIS WEEK

WHAT WAS THE BEST THING ABOUT THE WEEK?

MY RANKING OF THE WEEK

Daily Journal

Date:

Daily Journal

Date:

Daily Journal

Date:

Daily Journal

Date:

Daily Journal

Date:

Daily Journal

Date:

Daily Journal

Date:

Weekly check in

DATE _______________

Daily Journal

Date:

Daily Journal

Date:

Daily Journal

Date:

Daily Journal

Date:

Daily Journal

Date:

Daily Journal

Date:

Daily Journal

Date:

Weekly check in

TOP 3 THINGS I DID THIS WEEK

- ○ ______________________
- ○ ______________________
- ○ ______________________

THIS WEEK I FELT

NEXT WEEK I WANT TO

MOST REWARDING INTERACTION I HAD THIS WEEK

THINGS I ACCOMPLISHED THIS WEEK

WHAT WAS THE BEST THING ABOUT THE WEEK?

MY RANKING OF THE WEEK

☆ ☆ ☆ ☆ ☆

Daily Journal

Date:

Daily Journal

Date:

Daily Journal

Date:

Daily Journal

Date:

Daily Journal

Date:

Daily Journal

Date:

Daily Journal

Date:

Weekly check in

DATE _______________

TOP 3 THINGS I DID THIS WEEK

○ ___________________________

○ ___________________________

○ ___________________________

THIS WEEK I FELT

MOST REWARDING INTERACTION I HAD THIS WEEK

NEXT WEEK I WANT TO

____

____

____

____

THINGS I ACCOMPLISHED THIS WEEK

WHAT WAS THE BEST THING ABOUT THE WEEK?

MY RANKING OF THE WEEK
☆ ☆ ☆ ☆ ☆

Daily Journal

Date:

Daily Journal

Date:

Daily Journal

Date:

Daily Journal

Date:

Daily Journal

Date:

Daily Journal

Date:

Daily Journal

Date:

Weekly check in

DATE ___________

TOP 3 THINGS I DID THIS WEEK

○ __________________________________

○ __________________________________

○ __________________________________

THIS WEEK I FELT

NEXT WEEK I WANT TO

____

____

____

____

MOST REWARDING INTERACTION I HAD THIS WEEK

THINGS I ACCOMPLISHED THIS WEEK

WHAT WAS THE BEST THING ABOUT THE WEEK?

MY RANKING OF THE WEEK

☆ ☆ ☆ ☆ ☆

Daily Journal

Date:

Daily Journal

Date:

Daily Journal

Date:

Daily Journal

Date:

Daily Journal

Date:

Daily Journal

Date:

Daily Journal

Date:

Weekly check in

DATE _______________

TOP 3 THINGS I DID THIS WEEK
- ○ _______________
- ○ _______________
- ○ _______________

THIS WEEK I FELT

NEXT WEEK I WANT TO

MOST REWARDING INTERACTION I HAD THIS WEEK

THINGS I ACCOMPLISHED THIS WEEK

WHAT WAS THE BEST THING ABOUT THE WEEK?

MY RANKING OF THE WEEK
☆ ☆ ☆ ☆ ☆

Daily Journal

Date:

Daily Journal

Date:

Daily Journal

Date:

Daily Journal

Date:

Daily Journal

Date:

Daily Journal

Date:

Daily Journal

Date:

Weekly check in

DATE _______________

TOP 3 THINGS I DID THIS WEEK

1. _______________
2. _______________
3. _______________

THIS WEEK I FELT

NEXT WEEK I WANT TO

____
____
____
____

MOST REWARDING INTERACTION I HAD THIS WEEK

THINGS I ACCOMPLISHED THIS WEEK

WHAT WAS THE BEST THING ABOUT THE WEEK?

MY RANKING OF THE WEEK

☆ ☆ ☆ ☆ ☆

Daily Journal

Date:

Daily Journal

Date:

Daily Journal

Date:

Daily Journal

Date:

Daily Journal

Date:

Daily Journal

Date:

Daily Journal

Date:

Weekly check in

DATE _______________

TOP 3 THINGS I DID THIS WEEK

-
-
-

THIS WEEK I FELT

NEXT WEEK I WANT TO

MOST REWARDING INTERACTION I HAD THIS WEEK

THINGS I ACCOMPLISHED THIS WEEK

WHAT WAS THE BEST THING ABOUT THE WEEK?

MY RANKING OF THE WEEK

☆ ☆ ☆ ☆ ☆

Daily Journal

Date:

Daily Journal

Date:

Daily Journal

Date:

Daily Journal

Date:

Daily Journal

Date:

Daily Journal

Date:

Daily Journal

Date:

Weekly check in

DATE _______________

TOP 3 THINGS I DID THIS WEEK

○ _______________

○ _______________

○ _______________

THIS WEEK I FELT

NEXT WEEK I WANT TO

MOST REWARDING INTERACTION I HAD THIS WEEK

THINGS I ACCOMPLISHED THIS WEEK

WHAT WAS THE BEST THING ABOUT THE WEEK?

MY RANKING OF THE WEEK

☆ ☆ ☆ ☆ ☆

Daily Journal

Date:

Daily Journal

Date:

Daily Journal

Date:

Daily Journal

Date:

Daily Journal

Date:

Daily Journal

Date:

Daily Journal

Date:

Weekly check in

DATE

TOP 3 THINGS I DID THIS WEEK

- ○
- ○
- ○

THIS WEEK I FELT

NEXT WEEK I WANT TO

MOST REWARDING INTERACTION I HAD THIS WEEK

THINGS I ACCOMPLISHED THIS WEEK

WHAT WAS THE BEST THING ABOUT THE WEEK?

MY RANKING OF THE WEEK

Daily Journal

Date:

Daily Journal

Date:

Daily Journal

Date:

Daily Journal

Date:

Daily Journal

Date:

Daily Journal

Date:

Daily Journal

Date:

Weekly check in

DATE _______________

TOP 3 THINGS I DID THIS WEEK

- ○ _______________
- ○ _______________
- ○ _______________

THIS WEEK I FELT

NEXT WEEK I WANT TO

____
____
____
____

MOST REWARDING INTERACTION I HAD THIS WEEK

THINGS I ACCOMPLISHED THIS WEEK

WHAT WAS THE BEST THING ABOUT THE WEEK?

MY RANKING OF THE WEEK

Daily Journal

Date:

Daily Journal

Date:

Daily Journal

Date:

Daily Journal

Date:

Daily Journal

Date:

Daily Journal

Date:

Daily Journal

Date:

Weekly check in

DATE ______________

TOP 3 THINGS I DID THIS WEEK

○ ______________________

○ ______________________

○ ______________________

THIS WEEK I FELT

NEXT WEEK I WANT TO ______________

____

____

____

____

MOST REWARDING INTERACTION I HAD THIS WEEK

THINGS I ACCOMPLISHED THIS WEEK

WHAT WAS THE BEST THING ABOUT THE WEEK?

MY RANKING OF THE WEEK

Daily Journal

Date:

Daily Journal

Date:

Daily Journal

Date:

Daily Journal

Date:

Daily Journal

Date:

Daily Journal

Date:

Daily Journal

Date:

Weekly check in

TOP 3 THINGS I DID THIS WEEK

-
-
-

THIS WEEK I FELT

NEXT WEEK I WANT TO

____

____

____

____

MOST REWARDING INTERACTION I HAD THIS WEEK

THINGS I ACCOMPLISHED THIS WEEK

WHAT WAS THE BEST THING ABOUT THE WEEK?

MY RANKING OF THE WEEK

☆ ☆ ☆ ☆ ☆

Daily Journal

Date:

Daily Journal

Date:

Daily Journal

Date:

Daily Journal

Date:

Daily Journal

Date:

Daily Journal

Date:

Daily Journal

Date:

Weekly check in

DATE _______________

TOP 3 THINGS I DID THIS WEEK

- _______________
- _______________
- _______________

THIS WEEK I FELT

NEXT WEEK I WANT TO _______________

____

____

____

____

MOST REWARDING INTERACTION I HAD THIS WEEK

THINGS I ACCOMPLISHED THIS WEEK

WHAT WAS THE BEST THING ABOUT THE WEEK?

MY RANKING OF THE WEEK

Daily Journal

Date:

Daily Journal

Date:

Daily Journal

Date:

Daily Journal

Date:

Daily Journal

Date:

Daily Journal

Date:

Daily Journal

Date:

Weekly check in

TOP 3 THINGS I DID THIS WEEK

- ____________________
- ____________________
- ____________________

THIS WEEK I FELT

NEXT WEEK I WANT TO ____________________

____

____

____

____

MOST REWARDING INTERACTION I HAD THIS WEEK

THINGS I ACCOMPLISHED THIS WEEK

WHAT WAS THE BEST THING ABOUT THE WEEK?

MY RANKING OF THE WEEK

Daily Journal

Date:

Daily Journal

Date:

Daily Journal

Date:

Daily Journal

Date:

Daily Journal

Date:

Daily Journal

Date:

Daily Journal

Date:

Weekly check in

DATE _______________

TOP 3 THINGS I DID THIS WEEK

- ○ _______________
- ○ _______________
- ○ _______________

THIS WEEK I FELT

NEXT WEEK I WANT TO _______________

____

____

____

____

MOST REWARDING INTERACTION I HAD THIS WEEK

THINGS I ACCOMPLISHED THIS WEEK

WHAT WAS THE BEST THING ABOUT THE WEEK?

MY RANKING OF THE WEEK

☆ ☆ ☆ ☆ ☆

Daily Journal

Date:

Daily Journal

Date:

Daily Journal

Date:

Daily Journal

Date:

Daily Journal

Date:

Daily Journal

Date:

Daily Journal

Date:

Weekly check in

DATE _______________

TOP 3 THINGS I DID THIS WEEK

- _______________________________
- _______________________________
- _______________________________

THIS WEEK I FELT

NEXT WEEK I WANT TO

____
____
____
____

THINGS I ACCOMPLISHED THIS WEEK

MOST REWARDING INTERACTION I HAD THIS WEEK

WHAT WAS THE BEST THING ABOUT THE WEEK?

MY RANKING OF THE WEEK

Daily Journal

Date:

Daily Journal

Date:

Daily Journal

Date:

Daily Journal

Date:

Daily Journal

Date:

Daily Journal

Date:

Daily Journal

Date:

Weekly check in

DATE ___________

TOP 3 THINGS I DID THIS WEEK

○ _______________________

○ _______________________

○ _______________________

THIS WEEK I FELT

NEXT WEEK I WANT TO ___________

____

____

____

____

MOST REWARDING INTERACTION I HAD THIS WEEK

THINGS I ACCOMPLISHED THIS WEEK

WHAT WAS THE BEST THING ABOUT THE WEEK?

MY RANKING OF THE WEEK

Daily Journal

Date:

Daily Journal

Date:

Daily Journal

Date:

Daily Journal

Date:

Daily Journal

Date:

Daily Journal

Date:

Daily Journal

Date:

Weekly check in

DATE ___________

TOP 3 THINGS I DID THIS WEEK
-
-
-

THIS WEEK I FELT

NEXT WEEK I WANT TO

MOST REWARDING INTERACTION I HAD THIS WEEK

THINGS I ACCOMPLISHED THIS WEEK

WHAT WAS THE BEST THING ABOUT THE WEEK?

MY RANKING OF THE WEEK

Daily Journal

Date:

Daily Journal

Date:

Daily Journal

Date:

Daily Journal

Date:

Daily Journal

Date:

Daily Journal

Date:

Daily Journal

Date:

Weekly check in

DATE ______________

TOP 3 THINGS I DID THIS WEEK
○ ___________________________
○ ___________________________
○ ___________________________

THIS WEEK I FELT

NEXT WEEK I WANT TO

____
____
____
____

THINGS I ACCOMPLISHED THIS WEEK

MOST REWARDING INTERACTION I HAD THIS WEEK

WHAT WAS THE BEST THING ABOUT THE WEEK?

MY RANKING OF THE WEEK
☆ ☆ ☆ ☆ ☆

Daily Journal

Date:

Daily Journal

Date:

Daily Journal

Date:

Daily Journal

Date:

Daily Journal

Date:

Daily Journal

Date:

Daily Journal

Date:

Weekly check in

DATE ______________

TOP 3 THINGS I DID THIS WEEK

- ______________________________
- ______________________________
- ______________________________

THIS WEEK I FELT

NEXT WEEK I WANT TO ______________

____

____

____

____

THINGS I ACCOMPLISHED THIS WEEK

MOST REWARDING INTERACTION I HAD THIS WEEK

WHAT WAS THE BEST THING ABOUT THE WEEK?

MY RANKING OF THE WEEK

☆ ☆ ☆ ☆ ☆

Daily Journal

Date:

Daily Journal

Date:

Daily Journal

Date:

Daily Journal

Date:

Daily Journal

Date:

Daily Journal

Date:

Daily Journal

Date:

Weekly check in

DATE _______________

TOP 3 THINGS I DID THIS WEEK

○ _______________________

○ _______________________

○ _______________________

THIS WEEK I FELT

NEXT WEEK I WANT TO _______________

____

____

____

____

MOST REWARDING INTERACTION I HAD THIS WEEK

THINGS I ACCOMPLISHED THIS WEEK

WHAT WAS THE BEST THING ABOUT THE WEEK?

MY RANKING OF THE WEEK

Daily Journal

Date:

Daily Journal

Date:

Daily Journal

Date:

Daily Journal

Date:

Daily Journal

Date:

Daily Journal

Date:

Daily Journal

Date:

Weekly check in

DATE _______________

TOP 3 THINGS I DID THIS WEEK

- ___________________________
- ___________________________
- ___________________________

THIS WEEK I FELT

NEXT WEEK I WANT TO _______________

MOST REWARDING INTERACTION I HAD THIS WEEK

THINGS I ACCOMPLISHED THIS WEEK

WHAT WAS THE BEST THING ABOUT THE WEEK?

MY RANKING OF THE WEEK

☆ ☆ ☆ ☆ ☆

Daily Journal

Date:

Daily Journal

Date:

Daily Journal

Date:

Daily Journal

Date:

Daily Journal

Date:

Daily Journal

Date:

Daily Journal

Date:

Weekly check in

DATE __________

Daily Journal

Date:

Daily Journal

Date:

Daily Journal

Date:

Daily Journal

Date:

Daily Journal

Date:

Daily Journal

Date:

Daily Journal

Date:

Weekly check in

DATE ____________

TOP 3 THINGS I DID THIS WEEK

- ____________________
- ____________________
- ____________________

THIS WEEK I FELT

NEXT WEEK I WANT TO

MOST REWARDING INTERACTION I HAD THIS WEEK

THINGS I ACCOMPLISHED THIS WEEK

WHAT WAS THE BEST THING ABOUT THE WEEK?

MY RANKING OF THE WEEK

☆ ☆ ☆ ☆ ☆

Daily Journal

Date:

Daily Journal

Date:

Daily Journal

Date:

Daily Journal

Date:

Daily Journal

Date:

Daily Journal

Date:

Daily Journal

Date:

Weekly check in

DATE _______________

Daily Journal

Date:

Daily Journal

Date:

Daily Journal

Date:

Daily Journal

Date:

Daily Journal

Date:

Daily Journal

Date:

Daily Journal

Date:

Weekly check in

DATE _______________

TOP 3 THINGS I DID THIS WEEK

- ______________________________
- ______________________________
- ______________________________

THIS WEEK I FELT

MOST REWARDING INTERACTION I HAD THIS WEEK

NEXT WEEK I WANT TO

____
____
____
____

THINGS I ACCOMPLISHED THIS WEEK

WHAT WAS THE BEST THING ABOUT THE WEEK?

MY RANKING OF THE WEEK

Afterword

As you reach the closing pages of this journal, pause for a moment, and reflect upon the journey you've traversed. Within these pages, you've captured a year of dedication, resilience, challenges, and moments of profound connection. Every word you've written and every emotion you've expressed paints a unique portrait of love, patience, and commitment.

Caring for someone with dementia is a journey like no other. It challenges us in ways we never anticipated and teaches us lessons we might never have sought. Yet, amidst the tumultuous waves and calm seas, there lies a narrative of deep humanity, of connecting with another soul in their most vulnerable moments. Your journal entries are a testament to that.

It's my sincerest hope that this journal has provided a safe space for your thoughts and feelings. While caregiving can often feel isolating, remember you're never truly alone. We find community and connection through sharing stories, seeking support, and allowing ourselves to be vulnerable.

As you move forward, consider how this journaling experience has impacted you. Has it offered clarity during confusing times? Has it provided solace when you've needed it most? Perhaps it's been a faithful companion, ready to listen when the world seemed too loud or quiet.

Though the pages of this journal have been filled, your journey continues. It might be beneficial to revisit these pages occasionally as a remembrance and a source of strength and insight.

Finally, take a moment to acknowledge yourself. The very act of journaling, of taking time for introspection amidst your responsibilities, is an act of self-care and courage. You have taken steps, day by day, to ensure that your well-being is recognized and prioritized. Celebrate that.

From the depths of my heart, thank you for allowing this journal to accompany you. We wish you continued strength, abundant support, and moments of serenity in the days ahead.

With warmth and gratitude,

G. M. Grace

Your Next Essential Read
"Dementia Caregiver's Practical Guide"

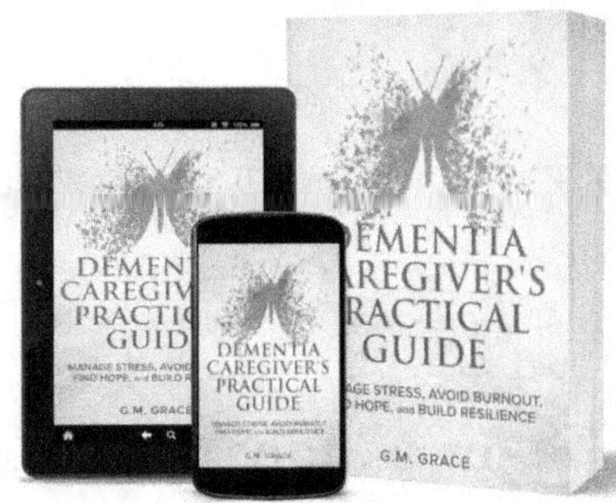

Are you looking to delve deeper into the world of dementia caregiving? To further equip yourself with practical knowledge, insights, and tools that can make your caregiving journey smoother?

We're delighted to introduce the "Dementia Caregiver's Practical Guide: Manage Stress, Avoid Burnout, Find Hope, and Build Resilience" — a comprehensive resource tailored for caregivers like you. Whether you're in the initial stages of understanding dementia or have been on this journey for some time, this guide promises valuable insights, techniques, and real-life solutions to the challenges faced by caregivers.

How to Access: We've incorporated a QR code on the next page for your convenience. Scan it with your smartphone or tablet, and it will lead you directly to the purchasing page for the "Dementia Caregiver's Practical Guide: Manage Stress, Avoid Burnout, Find Hope, and Build Resilience."

This seamless process ensures that the next step in your caregiving resource journey is just a scan away.

I genuinely believe in empowering caregivers with the best knowledge and support available. This guide is a testament to that belief. May it serve as a beacon of hope, clarity, and practical wisdom in your journey with your loved one.

Your Feedback Matters to Me!

I hope you are finding value in this journal. Your feedback is crucial to help me and others in this community of caregivers make informed choices. I would be deeply appreciative if you could spare a few minutes to share your thoughts and experiences on Amazon.

How to Leave a Review: Scan the QR code below using your smartphone or tablet's camera. This will direct you straight to the review page on Amazon. Share your honest feedback and rate the journal as per your experience.

Your insights not only help future readers/customers but also guide us in our mission to constantly improve and serve you better.